LITTLE-KNOWN SEX FACTS

Everything They Didn't Teach You in Sex Ed

LORENZO JENSEN III

Thought Catalog Books
Brooklyn, NY

THOUGHT CATALOG BOOKS

Copyright © 2015 by The Thought & Expression Co.

First edition, 2015
ISBN 978-1519740687
10 9 8 7 6 5 4 3 2 1

Founded in 2010, Thought Catalog is a website and imprint dedicated to your ideas and stories. We publish fiction and non-fiction from emerging and established writers across all genres.

Cover photography by © iStock.com/casarsa

CONTENTS

CHAPTER 1.

TWENTY-THREE WEIRD & DISTURBING SEX FACTS YOU REALLY DIDN'T NEED TO KNOW

---

1. Old people have a LOT of sex.

How much sex, you ask? Do you *really* want to know? OK, since you asked, the elderly are currently experiencing the biggest spike in sexually transmitted infections among all age groups. Should I continue? All right, then—three-quarters of 70-year-old men are still able to impregnate a woman. Should I stop? No? Then you need to know that nearly a third of women over 80 still have sex with their partners. And one-third of men and one-quarter of women over 50 have performed oral sex over the past year. Hey, don't blame me—you asked!

2. Female orgasm is designed to induce pregnancy.

The rhythmic pulsating motion of the vaginal walls during female orgasm is designed to push sperm up toward the uterus and into the cervix. And you thought the real purpose of the female orgasm was pleasure. How wrong you were!

3. The human mouth hosts over 500 types of bacteria.

Try not to think of that the next time you're kissing someone or they're going down on you. Visualizing 500 different types of bacteria squirming all over your junk could threaten to kill the mood.

4. Straight men comprise more than half the audience for online transgender porn.

A meta-study of one billion online searches for porn concluded that transgender porn is the fourth-most popular form of porn on Earth. And straight men are the primary consumers of it. There may actually be less transphobia out there than you think there is.

5. Left testicles tend to hang lower than right ones.

I'll pause to allow you to visually verify this fact with all your male friends—and I won't judge you for it!

6. Female penguins engage in a form of prostitution.

Researchers have repeatedly observed female penguins exchanging sexual favors with male penguins that aren't their mates in exchange for pebbles they will use to build nests for their babies.

7. Two-thirds of men and women have fantasized about other people while having sex with their partner.

Tonight when you're having sex with your partner, I want you both to fantasize that the other one is fantasizing about having sex with someone else. It's the only way to keep some spice in your love life.

8. Ovulating women are more likely to cheat.

When that egg's sitting there just *aching* to be fertilized, women tend to get a little restless.

And if you can't do the job, well, boy, you're fired.

9. Shaving your pubes makes you more likely to spread a sexually transmitted infection.

Since pubic hair acts as a sort of sexual hockey goalie, it is assumed that shaved pubes will also make it more likely for you to receive a sexually transmitted infection. Clearly this is God's way of showing us that it's time for everyone to end the madness and "go natural" again.

10. Male testosterone levels and sperm counts are only a quarter of what they were a century ago.

Men aren't what they used to be. In fact, they are literally only a quarter of what they used to be only a century ago.

11. Male fruit flies who can't find mates are more likely to drink alcohol than fruit flies who are players.

I have no idea where these fruit flies are getting alcohol—one would assume they'd at least be carded at the local bar—but fruit flies who are losers at the mating game tend to drown their misery in booze.

12. Alfred Kinsey was able to insert the bristle side of a toothbrush into his urethra.

The pioneering sex researcher and author of *The Kinsey Report* also had a collection of over 5,000 wasps. Why he was sticking toothbrushes up his urethra and collecting thousands of wasps is probably a problem for him and his therapist. Either way, it's pretty freaky-deaky.

13. Sex toys are banned in Alabama and Mississippi.

Can you fucking believe they make you drive to Georgia and Arkansas for sex toys? Gas isn't cheap, you know!

14. Women are aroused by chimpanzee porn.

That's right, as weeeeeeeird as that is. A study showed that women who viewed footage of chimpanzee sex became sexually aroused and experienced vaginal lubrication.

15. Four popes have died while having sex.

Sure, that means that 262 popes did *not* die during sex, but these are *popes*—they're not supposed to be having sex in the first place.

16. Adults are more likely to tell lies while in bed than they are anywhere else.

This is really hard to believe, since you're usually naked in bed and it's hard to exaggerate *anything* in that condition. But people lie more when they're lying in bed—get it?

17. Gay men have bigger penises than straight men.

Although straight men tend to be bigger dicks.

18. The bigger his balls, the more likely he is to cheat.

If your man has huge testes, the only sane thing to do is get a GPS tracking chip implanted in his body while he's sleeping—that way you'll always know where he is.

19. Educated white women have more anal sex than any other group.

This presumably includes educated white gay men. Uh—way to go, white women?

20. Fat men have more sexual endurance than thin men.

Multiple studies have confirmed that it takes severely overweight men nearly three times as long to ejaculate as it does those jerky male gym rats who are always asking you to feel their six-packs. Six-packs? More like six seconds!

21. Male bicyclists risk impotence.

The pressure of the bicycle seat on the male groin can permanently damage sexual function and render the avid cyclist a poor and pathetic shell of his former sexual self. Is it really worth it? Drive a car instead and save your boners, guys!

22. Straight men search for images of penises online almost as much as they do vaginas.

It's unclear whether they're comparing themselves to the online penises or they simply like looking at them. If it's the latter, it raises the question of exactly how "straight" they really are.

23. One out of every ten European babies is conceived on an IKEA bed.

Just knowing this fact will make me unable to have an erection for three days. I hate IKEA.

CHAPTER 2.

BONING UP ON BONERS: TWENTY-THREE VEINY, THROBBING FACTS ABOUT ERECTIONS

---

1. JUST LIKE HEARTS, PENISES CAN BE BROKEN

Even though there is technically no "bone" in a "boner," it can still break during rough sex—and it even makes a horrible snapping noise! *OUCH!* During what is known variously as a "broken penis" or a "penile fracture"—which happens to an estimated 200 unfortunate American men yearly, and often while a woman is riding them on top—blood vessels explode, the penis swells and becomes dark purple, and your little willy is out of commission for at least six weeks because it's stuck at home in bed wearing a tiny penis splint.

2. MOST MAMMALS HAVE LITERAL BONERS

Along with horses, *Homo sapiens* is one of the few mammals whose "boners" don't literally contain bones.

3. IT HAS A MIND OF ITS OWN

Your penis is ruled by your autonomic nervous system, much like your heart rate and blood pressure. That means that sexual arousal is often involuntary and occurs at the most humiliating times, as any teenage boy with a raging erection who's had to deliver a lecture on snails in the front of the entire ninth-grade biology class can attest.

4. THREE KINDS OF BONERS

Scientists who spend a lot of time thinking about boners and measuring them—I would guess they're called "erectologists"—break down erections into three categories: 1) psychogenic (the result of fantasies); 2) reflexogenic (the result of physical stimulation; and 3) nocturnal (the result of getting an involuntary hard-on while you're passed out cold and snoring like a crocodile).

5. FOUR BLOODY SHOTS OF WHISKEY

In order to make the miraculous transition from flaccid to hard, the average human penis must fill with four whiskey shots worth of blood. Then again, if you also *drink* four whiskey shots, you may have trouble getting hard at all.

6. MEN ARE 'ROUND-THE-CLOCK ERECTION MACHINES

Whether awake or asleep, most men average 11 erections every day—that's from when the cock crows until the cock crows again the next morning.

7. FETUSES HAVE BONERS, TOO

The developers of ultrasound technology probably didn't expect that their invention would reveal that male fetuses start getting erections during their third trimester in the womb, and now that you're aware of this fact, you will never be able to wipe it from your brain.

8. BONERS AFTER DEATH

Men who die via hanging are prone to getting a "death erection" when gravity forces blood down into their penile tissue. This phenomenon is known as "angel lust."

9. ORGASMS WITHOUT ERECTIONS

Yes, it happens—some men can have orgasms without ever getting even slightly hard. This probably makes them happy. Their partners? Not so much.

10. HALF OF IT IS INSIDE YOUR BODY

If your penis measures five inches, you can tell people it's ten inches, because that's technically true. Half of your penis will always be concealed inside your body, and you can feel it while you're erect if you press down on your perineum, AKA your "taint." There's the rest of your boner, tucked safely inside of you.

11. THE POISONOUS SPIDER THAT KILLS ERECTILE DYSFUNCTION

The Brazilian wandering spider wanders around Brazil inflicting tremendous suffering upon humans—but there's also an upside! The spider's toxic venom can induce priapism in men, which means that while they're writhing around on the floor due to loss of muscle control, they will also enjoy a robust hard-on while they're doing it.

12. ERECTIONS LASTING LONGER THAN FOUR HOURS

Priapism is a medical condition in which the penis stays as hard as a lead pipe for at least four hours and steadfastly refuses to soften. It doesn't sound bad to your run-of-the-mill premature ejaculator who can barely last once it's out of his pants, but priapism can be an extremely painful condition that can ultimately result in the loss of one's penis.

13. IF YOU WANT A BETTER BONER, STOP TOUCHING YOURSELF!

Guys, studies have shown that when you quit playing with yourself all the goddamn time, blood flow increases to your penis during those rare occasions when you might actually be having sex with someone else. So for the sake of your partner—and for God's sake as well—stop touching yourself all the time.

14. A BLOW-UP BALLOON BETWEEN YOUR LEGS

If you should suffer the tragic misfortune of not only being unable to achieve an erection by yourself, but you find that even tried-and-true boner pills such as Viagra and Cialis don't do the trick, you can always get a penile implant. Whenever you want to get hard, you just pump a little grape-sized valve that's been implanted in your scrotum, and your limp dick will inflate like a party balloon within seconds! It only involves an extensive surgery that places plastic rods inside your penile shaft and a reservoir of saline solution in your stomach, and there's nothing about any of this which should make you self-conscious or your female partner nauseated!

15. MEDICATIONS THAT CAUSE IMPOTENCE

If you're taking Adderall, antidepressants, antihistamines, diet pills, and/or tranquilizers, you might have to kiss that erection of yours goodbye, because all of these medications are extremely boner-hostile.

16. LIVE FAST, LOSE YOUR ERECTION

Certain unsavory lifestyle choices—such as smoking tobacco or weed, snorting meth or cocaine, shooting heroin, and alcohol abuse—can cause nerve damage, shrink your testicles, lower your testosterone levels, soften your erection, and cause you to lose your girlfriend.

17. MEASURE FROM THE TOP SIDE

If you'd like to measure your erection—and it's a verified scientific fact that every young man in world history has done it multiple times—measure it from your tummy side, not from your scrotum side. Leave the scrotum side alone. It's gross down there.

18. GROWERS V. SHOWERS

A "grower" penis is one that increases significantly in size when it becomes erect. A "shower" is one you show off when it's limp, because it doesn't get that much bigger when hard. Research has shown that shorter penises expand around 86% when they get hard, as opposed to longer ones, which grow only about 47%.

19. THIRTY MILLION MALFUNCTIONING AMERICAN PENISES

Around 30 million American men suffer the heartache and humiliation of erectile dysfunction, also known as "ED," which is probably the most annoying acronym in the world to guys named Ed.

20. RECORD FOR CONSECUTIVE EJACULATIONS WITHOUT GOING SOFT

The official world record for consecutive male orgasms without loss of one's erection is a staggering six blown wads over the span of thirty-six minutes without once going soft. Bravo, señor!

21. ERECTIONS NEED EXERCISE

If you don't have regular erections, your penis muscles will atrophy just as your biceps will if you aren't regularly lifting weights. Without a steady diet of boners, your penis can lose up to an inch in length—and you don't want that, do you?

22. RIDE THE LIGHTNING

Nitric oxide is caused naturally by lightning. Nitric oxide is also the chemical compound that increases blood flow to the penis and causes erections so sturdy, they may as well be lightning rods.

23. PURPLE HOMEWRECKER?

Euphemisms for "erection" include boner, hard-on, woodie, stiffie, pocket rocket, chubbie, throbbing gristle, and purple homewrecker.

CHAPTER 3.

FIFTEEN FUN AND FREAKY FACTS ABOUT FORESKINS

---

1. HELP! THERE'S A BABY FORESKIN IN MY FACIAL CREAM!

While you may have assumed that circumcised foreskins languish in a hospital dumpster before being eternally consigned to a landfill, the medical and cosmetics industries swoop down like buzzards on these discarded penile skin flaps and make money by using them to heal wrinkles and burns.

Newborn foreskins contain human growth factors that make them ideal for anti-wrinkle skin creams. Face creams that use baby foreskins include SkinMedica and HydraFacial.

Baby foreskins are roughly the size of a postage stamp—yes, I guess someone actually took the time to measure one—but "can grow to the size of three basketball courts in less than a month" under the proper laboratory conditions. The skin is then used for grafts to aid in the healing of burn victims.

2. WOMEN HAVE FORESKINS, TOO

What is known as the "foreskin" in males is called the "clitoral hood" in females. Both are designed to protect these pleasure centers from harm. If gender-neutral is your thang, both foreskins and clitoral hoods are known as prepuces.

3. THE 4,400-YEAR-OLD FORESKIN

An Egyptian bas-relief from 2400 B.C. depicts a flint-knife circumcision and is thought to be the earliest historical mention of foreskin removal.

4. OVER 100 AMERICAN MALE INFANTS DIE FROM CIRCUMCISION YEARLY

On average, 117 American boys die yearly from post-circumcision complications, most of them involving blood loss or infections.

5. MORE FORESKIN = MORE PLEASURE

The average male foreskin contains 20,000 nerve endings. According to one study, the *least* sensitive part of the foreskin is *more* sensitive than the rest of the penis. During intercourse, the foreskin produces a "gliding action" that reduces friction and enhances lubrication. On the downside, having a foreskin feels so good that uncut men are more likely to develop premature ejaculation, a condition which will always be hilarious regardless of context.

6. PRO-FORESKIN ACTIVISTS CALL THEMSELVES 'INTACTIVISTS'

According to an anti-circumcision group called Bloodstained Men, an "intactivist" is:

> Someone who believes that every child, regardless of their gender or parents' beliefs, has the right to their intact genitals, as they're born.

Other groups that see circumcision as a barbaric, unnecessary, and nonconsensual mutilation of infant genitals are Brothers United for Future Foreskins (BUFF) and National Organization of Restoring Men (NORM).

7. HAVING A FORESKIN CAN LEAD TO MEDICAL PROBLEMS...

According to Dr. Brian Morris of the University of Sydney, uncircumcised men are fifty times more likely to develop penile cancer than men who've been "cut."

Intact foreskins contain what are known as Langerhans cells, which facilitate HIV transmission. As a result, uncircumcised men are 60% more likely to acquire HIV than men who've been snipped.

Uncircumcised men can also develop a condition called phimosis in which the foreskin envelops the penis too tightly, which can lead to urine getting trapped in the foreskin and turning the entire shlong into a swollen pee balloon.

8. ...BUT SO CAN BEING CIRCUMCISED

Men who've been circumcised are nearly five times as likely to develop erectile dysfunction as those who've never undergone the tortures and torments of postpartum penile mutilation. They are also said to be 60% more likely to develop a psychological disorder known as alexithymia, which makes it difficult to express one's emotions.

9. SOME GIRLS HATE 'EM

On an episode of *Seinfeld*, Elaine admits to sleeping with an uncircumcised man. "It had no face, no personality," she kvetches about his penis.

According to one woman, "I believe uncircumcised penises have a very off-putting odor!" Another says, "I've found that uncircumcised penises tend to have a stronger smell and more greasy/sweaty feel to them."

10. SOME GIRLS LOVE 'EM

One US study found that 85% of women who'd had sex with both cut and uncut men preferred men with foreskins. One of the main reasons they offered is that foreskins aid in the production of that nasty excretory paste known as smegma, which acts as a natural lubricant.

Other women find cut penises to be visually revolting: "I think circumcised penises look like mutilated, skinned mushrooms, and there's that ugly scar on it," gripes one foreskin-lovin' lass.

11. THERE WAS A PUNK BAND CALLED 'THE 4-SKINS"

The 4-Skins were a quartet of London East Enders who played Oi! Music and were associated with the skinhead scene. I never met them, so I cannot confirm whether any of them retained their foreskins into adulthood.

12. THE INVENTOR OF CORN FLAKES RECOMMENDED SEWING BOYS' FORESKINS SHUT

John Harvey Kellogg—he of cereal fame—was intensely concerned about the fact that boys and girls all across America were furiously masturbating without his consent and approval. One of the methods he recommended for discouraging masturbation among uncircumcised boys was sewing their foreskins shut with a metal wire.

13. THE QUEST FOR THE HOLY FORESKIN

Throughout much of the Christian era, rumors spread through Europe of a "Holy Foreskin" that had been clipped from Jesus at birth. The first reported Holy Foreskin sighting was in 800 A.D. when Emperor Charlemagne bequeathed the alleged divine prepuce to the Pope. According to an expert on Catholic relics, "Depending on what you read, there were eight, twelve, fourteen, or even 18 different holy foreskins in various European towns during the Middle Ages." Perhaps they'd been multiplying like fishes and loaves. Embarrassed by the whole topic, in the year 1900 Pope Leo XIII ordered the immediate excommunication of any Catholic who even mentioned the Holy Foreskin.

14. TUGGING YOUR WAY BACK TO SQUARE ONE

Foreskin restoration is all the rage among men who feel that they were cruelly, painfully, and unnecessarily mutilated as infants by a foreskin-phobic society. This can be accomplished surgically by using skin from the scrotum, which everyone can agree is an ugly human body part with an exceedingly ugly name. For those who prefer to take the natural route, a sometimes years-long process of stretching the skin both manually and with weights is known as "tugging."

15. THE RABBI, THE WALLET, AND THE SUITCASE

There's an old joke about a rabbi who keeps

all the foreskins from circumcisions he's performed and makes them into a wallet. The rabbi's friend remarks that it seems like he went through an awful lot of trouble just to make a wallet. "I know," the rabbi replies, "but when you rub it, it turns into a suitcase."

CHAPTER 4.

TWENTY-FIVE LITTLE-KNOWN FACTS ABOUT PENISES

---

1. What you see is only half of what you've got.

Unfortunately, half of your penis is tucked away inside your body and attached to the pubic bone.

2. Your penis is crawling with bacteria.

Researchers in Arizona found 42 types of bacteria on men's penises. That's 42 more types than are acceptable.

3. It takes over four ounces of blood to achieve an erection.

One would assume that blood comes straight from the brain.

4. Penis size is not correlated to shoe size.

So put away your clown shoes. You're not fooling anyone.

5. Penises stop growing in your early 20s.

In other words, your penis stops growing right when you start growing up.

6. A man's penis is never bigger than when he's receiving oral sex.

A scientific study determined that men's penises measure the largest during a right good blowjob.

7. Smoking can make your penis smaller.

You may think it looks cool to smoke, but you'll look a lot less cool once you drop your drawers.

8. Four-fifths of men are "growers"; the rest are "showers."

Most men's penises grow much larger when they get an erection. The rest really don't improve much in size at all. Sucks to be them.

9. Bigger penises may be an evolutionary advantage.

This is because longer penises are better able to flush out a rival's sperm. If you want to know why she was fucking a rival in the first place, you'd better ask her.

10. Only 6% of men require an extra-large condom.

Although probably half of them buy them anyway.

11. Penises are usually darker than the rest of your body.

And it has nothing to do with anal sex.

12. If you don't use it, you might lose it.

Inactivity can shrink the penis from 1-2 centimeters, so start jerking off again immediately.

13. The underside is the most sensitive part.

Are you taking notes, ladies?

14. Penises lose sensation with age.

But by then you're too senile to notice.

15. Globally, less than a third of men are circumcised.

Although nearly two-thirds of American men are circumcised.

16. Most men think they're smaller than they actually are.

Even though they might brag that they're bigger than they actually are.

17. Fetuses can have erections.

Well, c'mon—you're in there for nine months. It gets boring after a while. You have to do *something* to kill the time.

18. It is almost impossible to achieve an erection in outer space.

This is according to astronauts' personal testimonials.

19. There's a reason his looks bigger than yours.

Well, one reason may be that it's actually bigger. But the angle from which a man views his own penis makes it appear smaller than an identically sized penis when viewed on another.

20. Some men have two penises.

About 100 men in the world, to be exact. The condition is known as "diphallus."

21. Hanging victims often achieve erections.

But the "being dead" part makes it impossible to enjoy them.

22. The smallest human penis ever recorded was 5/8 of an inch.

Weep for that poor fellow, will you?

23. The smallest animal penis is 1/5 of an inch.

And it belongs to the male shrew. So tell me again why they need to be tamed?

24. The penis has no muscles.

Instead it's more like a sponge, except sponges aren't nearly as pleasurable.

25. During missionary position, penises assume a boomerang shape.

MRI evidence confirms this. Why that dude was using an MRI during sex is anyone's guess.

CHAPTER 5.

TWENTY-THREE LITTLE-KNOWN FACTS ABOUT ORGASMS

---

1. A select few lucky individuals are able to reach orgasm simply by thinking.

And I think I'm jealous of those people. In fact, I know I am.

2. About one in ten women can reach orgasm merely by exercising.

This is known variously as the "yogasm," the "coregasm," and the "iwishthiswouldhappen-tomegasm."

3. Having an orgasm can burn calories.

OK, so it's only 2-3 calories, so you'll have to cum about 100 times for every donut you eat.

4. Up to 94% of women in one study say they can achieve orgasm via anal penetration.

This is a much higher quotient than women who can achieve it through vaginal penetration, so maybe it's time guys considered becoming a "back door man."

5. Wearing high heels may negatively affect a woman's orgasmic pleasure.

Researchers speculate that this is because during orgasm, a woman's feet curl to roughly the same shape as when she's wearing high heels, so if she's already wearing them, this diminishes her pleasure.

6. A minority of women have orgasms during childbirth.

But it's probably wise not to tell their children if they did.

7. Men think women cum more often than women actually do.

The so-called "orgasm gap" refers to one study where 85% of men said they thought their female partner came, while only 64% of those women say they actually did.

8. Orgasms can actually relieve pain.

But only for about 8-10 minutes, at which it's time to have another orgasm or pop another Percocet.

9. It seems like a "pain face," but it's actually an "orgasm face."

People in the throes of sexual ecstasy often look like they're in pain because orgasm activates the same brain regions that pain activates. Either that, or their partner accidentally kneed them in the groin while they were cumming.

10. Cum often, live longer.

A study in the *British Medical Journal* reports that men between the ages of 45-59 who have fewer than two orgasms a week are twice as likely to die than men who are wantonly squirting their filthy juices all over the place.

11. Women have "wet dreams," too.

One study found that over a third of women reported that at least once in their lives, they'd had orgasms while asleep.

12. For men, having an orgasm is like taking a shot of heroin.

One Danish study revealed that when men have an orgasm, it lights up the same brain centers that get let when heroin users shoot up. No wonder so many men become sex addicts.

13. Men fake orgasm, too.

According to a University of Kansas study of male college students, over a quarter of them confessed to faking orgasm at least once. Many said it was because they were too drunk to cum; others said they were merely tired and wanted to get some sleep.

14. Men need time to rest between orgasms, while women don't.

And you never let us hear the end of it, especially if you're naturally loud in the sack.

15. The most sexually satisfied women are over age 80.

And it is to be assumed that their partners are not men over age 80.

16. The bigger his belly, the smaller his load.

Fellas, if your Body Mass Index is over 30, it is highly likely that the amount of your ejaculate will be only half as much as those of us who take care of ourselves and have bitchin' abs.

17. Women take longer than men to cum.

On average, men require between two and ten minutes before they shoot their wad and start snoring. Women take twenty minutes on average to cum, which presumably happens after that selfish asshole is already snoring.

18. Because of this, men need to engage in foreplay.

Guys, you need to do more than stick it, shoot it, and start snoring. You need to kiss her. Rub her nipples. Gently lick her. Tell her you love her whether it's true or not. Her sexuality is far more complicated than your own, which is roughly as complicated as that of a brain-dead reptile.

19. Up to a fifth of American women have never had an orgasm.

This is a national crisis greater than poverty, terrorism, and the Kardashians combined.

20. You are more likely to be robbed or attacked directly after an orgasm.

I'm not saying anything about your partner, it's just that the brain areas that are attuned to fear and danger shut down temporarily directly subsequent to an orgasm, making you more vulnerable to a criminal assault.

21. A woman's orgasmic contractions pulsate in opposite directions depending on her menstrual cycle.

During menstruation, a woman's orgasmic contractions push outward to push all "waste," including male sperm, out of her body. During ovulation, the contractions have an inward motion in order to suck sperm upward toward her uterus.

22. Men have "G" spots, too.

In a stroke of cruel genius, God placed it about two inches up their butts.

23. Night of the living dead orgasms.

Researchers have determined that whose who are legally brain-dead but whose hearts are still beating are able to achieve sexual climax when given proper stimulation. This is known as the "Lazarus reflex," which is more than I already needed to know.

CHAPTER 6.

TWENTY LITTLE-KNOWN FACTS ABOUT NIPPLES

---

1. Your nipples and your earlobes are spaced apart exactly the same.

Check in the mirror if you don't believe me.

2. Pink nipple makeup is all the rage in Japan.

The Japanese, bless their souls, are in the throes of pink-nipple mania. Since Asian nipples tend to be browner, there's a whole cottage industry where women use makeup to render their nips pinker.

3. No two nipples are alike—just like snowflakes!

Even your own nipples are different from one another. Diversity is a strength!

4. The left one is usually more sensitive.

"Erotic sensitivity" of the nipples is more commonly intense on the left side. Correspondingly, nearly two-thirds of women have a larger left breast than a right one.

5. Some people are born with no nipples.

The condition is known as "athelia," and there are only about 7,000 diagnosed cases worldwide.

6. Some people are born with triple nipples—or more!

Any nipples beyond two on a human being are known as "supernumerary" nipples. One in every 18 males and one in every 50 women has more than two nipples. This means that there are over 27 million Americans with supernumerary nipples. Mark Wahlberg has three. Harry Styles has four. In 2012, a man in India was found to have seven nipples. In the Middle Ages, anyone with more than two nipples was thought to be demon-possessed. It was also thought that the Devil sucked from their triple nipples. The Devil is a stone-cold freak!

7. Innies v. Outies.

An estimated 10 to 20 percent of women have "inverted nipples," which means instead of protruding, they actually sink below the areola. They are also known as "shy nipples."

8. Nipplegasms.

Nipple stimulation affects the same part of the brain as genital stimulation does. A tiny minority of women are able to reach orgasm solely through having their nips caressed.

9. Some nipples get darker during sexual arousal.

This is caused by a rush of blood to the area during sexual stimulation.

10. Then again, maybe she's just cold.

Although erect nipples can be sign of sexual arousal, they also can get hard merely because it's too cold. So before you misinterpret her rock-hard nips as a sign that she's ready to rut, make sure that drafty window isn't open.

11. Those little bumps on the areola are called Montgomery glands.

These glands were first described in an 1837 scientific paper by William Montgomery. They secrete a white lubricant for the skin, but the reason for their existence remains unclear otherwise.

12. Everyone's nipples are hairy.

You may not be able to see them with the naked eye, but if you dare grab a magnifying glass and examine, you will find hairs growing on the areola of all adult living human beings.

13. Nipples start developing in the womb before sex organs do.

This is why both men and women have nipples—because they develop in the womb before sexual differentiation does.

14. "The Great Nippulini" has the world's strongest nipples.

Sage "The Great Nippulini" Werbock has built a career as a "nipple strongman." His dynamic feats of nipple strength include pulling a 2,200-pound vehicle 66 feet with his nipples. Whatever floats your boat, dude!

15. Some women in Asia suffer from the fear that their nipples will be suddenly sucked into their breasts.

Throughout Africa and Asia, "koro" is a psychological syndrome wherein males dread that their penises will disappear. The female version involves a morbid fear that their nipples will suddenly sink into their breasts, never to be seen again.

16. The nipple-licking drug gangs of Thailand.

In the late 1990s, it was discovered that Thailand's drug gangs had a widespread practice of having female members smear knockout drugs over their nipples. They would then seduce tourists and ask them to lick their nipples. The tourists would then pass out and be robbed of all their earthly belongings, as well as a huge chunk of their pride.

17. Are you Irish? Then go suck the king's nipples.

The ancient Irish considered their king's nipples to be sacred. During royal ceremonies, it was customary for his underlings to suck on his nipples. In power struggles, an opponent's nipples were often mutilated to prevent them from ever ascending to the throne.

18. Men and infants can lactate.

Newborn infants have been observed with milk leaking from their nipples. It only lasts for a few days. Adult men, especially if they've received hormone treatments for prostate cancer, have also been known to excrete milk through their nipples.

19. Nipple cancer is known as Paget's disease.

Affecting only the areola and nipple, Paget's disease accounts for between one and four percent of all breast-cancer cases.

20. There's even a word for having nipples.

That word is "mammillated." Nearly all human beings are mammillated at least twice over.

CHAPTER 7.

FIFTEEN LITTLE-KNOWN FACTS ABOUT PUBIC HAIR

---

1. The longest pubic hair in history was 28 inches.

A woman named Maoni Vi from Cape Town, South Africa had a pubic hair that measured 28 inches. She also had an armpit hair that measured 32 inches.

2. In Asia, women pay for pubic hair transplants.

As opposed to the West, where women are relentlessly pube-shamed and are always waxing themselves to the point where their external genitals are as smooth as a baby seal, Asian women—particularly those in South Korea—pay top dollar to have pubic hair implanted onto their crotches to give them that fuller, lusher, more natural look.

3. Pubic wigs are a thing.

These genital toupees—formally known as "merkins"—were thought to be first introduced in the 1400s as a means for prostitutes to cover up signs of STDs. They were also popular in the sexually repressed Victorian era. These days—when shearing one's natural wool is all the rage—sometimes actors will wear merkins if they're trying to recreate "period pieces," pun partially intended.

4. There's a biological reason the carpet doesn't always match the drapes.

If a person's pubic hair is a different color than the hair on their scalp, it may not be due to the fact that they're dying either area. Hair color is determined by the amount of melanin in the area where the hair is growing, which is why one's pubic hair is almost always darker than the hair on their head—because there's more melanin around your crotch than on your scalp.

5. Pubic balding is also a thing.

Medical conditions such as menopause, alopecia, an underactive adrenal gland, and cirrhosis of the liver can cause pubic hair to fall out. You may not have to pay for painful Brazilian waxes and expensive laser hair removal after all!

6. The weird history of pubic-hair souvenirs.

The British upper crust of the 1700s and 1800s had an odd habit of collecting the pubic hair of one's lovers as a souvenir—or, if you will, a hunting trophy. Scotland's St. Andrews University has a museum containing a snuff-box that is stuffed to the gills with the pubes of a mistress of King George IV. Other men of the era would attach their lover's pubic hair onto their hats as a public display of their sexual prowess.

7. You had hair on your genitals as a kid—you just couldn't see it.

What is known as "vellus hair"—thin, fine tufts that are nearly visible to the naked eye—is present on all children. What is known as "pubic hair" is the coarser, curlier, bushier hair that appears during the onset of adolescence.

8. There's actually a technical term for the onset of pubic hair during adolescence.

That term is "pubarche." I can see that word being repurposed as a synonym for "douchebag." Yeah, that guy was acting like a *total* pubarche last night.

9. The first major adult magazine to show a full-on bush was *Playboy* in 1971.

Although "smut" rags and still photos have featured full-blown "disco bushes" since photography was invented, the first major adult mag to show a healthy, vibrant, lush, exotic, three-dimensional female bush was during Liv Lindeland's *Playboy* pictorial of January 1971.

10. The strange case of the 16-month-old Alabama infant with adult public hair.

A 2007 issue of *Clinical Pediatrics* details the case of a 16-month-old Alabama boy with full pubic-hair development and an adult-sized penis. It turned out that his father had been prescribed testosterone gel, which he'd smear all over his body before climbing into bed and cuddling with his newborn. The excess testosterone induced an *extremely* premature adolescence in the male infant.

11. Missouri has a pubic-waxing law for minors.

In Missouri, children under 18 are forbidden from being waxed "on or near genitalia" unless they provide proof of parental consent.

12. Why it's curly.

Under a microscope, pubic hair is flat in shape like linguine. It is similar to African scalp hair in configuration, which causes it to curl when it reaches a certain length. In contrast, long, straight hair looks is shaped round like spaghetti when viewed under a microscope.

13. Female pubes popped up all over the place in famous paintings of the 1800s.

This includes Katsushika Hokusai's *The Dream of the Fisherman's Wife* (1813), Francisco Goya's *La Maja Desnuda* (circa 1800), and Gustave Courbet's *L'Origin Du Monde* (1866), which features a bush so lush, you could plant tomatoes in it.

14. But one art critic of the 1800s allegedly divorced his newlywed wife when he discovered that she rocked a bush.

Art critic John Ruskin must not have been paying attention to all those famous paintings of female pubes during the 1800s, because according to a biographer, he thought his wife was "a monster" on his wedding night when she revealed a natural bush instead of the marble-smooth mons pubis one sees in ancient sculptures of women.

15. Pubic hairs are exchanged during sex.

If you and your partner both have pubic hair, chances are that you will swap a few stray pubes during intercourse. Hey, it's better than transmitting an STD or inducing an unwanted pregnancy, right?

CHAPTER 8.

TWENTY-FIVE LITTLE-KNOWN FACTS ABOUT VAGINAS

---

1. Fear not—it's only a hole.

Technically, the "vagina" is a hole surrounded by the rest of the female genitalia, which includes the vaginal muscles, the cervix, the uterus, the labia, and the clitoris. But for the sake of convenience, nearly everyone refers to all of the female genitalia as the "vagina," so we will, too.

2. That hole is only about 3.5 inches deep.

In its resting state, the vagina is barely large enough to contain your house keys.

3. But that hole can become twice as deep during arousal.

Like the male organ, the vagina can double in size when it's sexually aroused, enabling it to contain at least two sets of house keys.

4. The clitoris contains about 8,000 nerve endings.

By contrast, the much larger penis head boasts a mere 3,500 nerve endings, although the entire penis contains about 24,000 nerve endings.

5. The word "vagina" comes from a Latin term meaning "sword holder."

Goddamned patriarchy, making everything about penises—even vaginas.

6. Vaginas share something special with...a shark's liver?

A compound known as squalane acts as a vaginal lubricant. It is also found in shark livers. (Cue every man in America asking their butcher if they carry shark livers.)

7. The vagina's pH level is similar to that of beer, wine, and tomatoes.

The average vagina has a pH level of 4, which qualifies as acidic. Sperm has a pH level of 8, which is basic, but you already knew that most guys are basic.

8. Pubic hair is sexual bait.

Some researchers speculate that pubic hair serves as a pheromone trap that lures the unsuspecting mate toward it much like the scent of pancakes grilling on a sunny summer morn.

9. Pubic hair only grows for three weeks.

Whereas the hair on your head can grow for up to seven years, your pubic hair will never get so long that you can lose your iPhone in it.

10. Only a minority of women get vaginal orgasms.

Only about one quarter of women are able to achieve orgasm strictly through intercourse, which is why youse guys need to pay extra attention to her love button.

11. What you eat affects how it smells.

Go easy on the garlic-and-sardines sandwiches and nibble on some pineapple chunks with strawberries instead.

12. Your discharge will change consistency during ovulation.

During ovulation, cervical mucus becomes clear and rubbery, just like your boyfriend's brain.

13. Unlike your roommates, your vagina cleans itself.

Therefore, there is no need to douche. Actually, douching can throw off your vagina's delicate bacterial balance and create a tragic situation between your legs. Only a douche would tell you to douche.

14. It can fall out of your body.

OK, it doesn't fall *entirely* out and splat onto the floor, but "vaginal prolapse" is a real condition wherein the vagina plops outside of the vulva and hangs down like a sock.

15. The mysterious "G" spot may actually be the underside of the clitoris.

Although debate persists on whether the "G" spot actually exists, some evidence suggests it's merely a sensitive area connected to the deep underside of your clitoris.

16. Vaginal farts are common.

Nearly all women get them. Take pride rather than shame in this fact. Hell, you can even form a lady's chorus where you queef in harmony like individual pipes in a pipe organ.

17. Being morally "loose" will not make your vagina loose.

The vagina is elastic like a rubber band, so no matter how many donkey shows you perform in Tijuana, it will snap back to its regular shape after sex.

18. On the flip side, abstinence will not make the vagina grow tighter.

Now you can take even less comfort in being celibate.

19. Unlike sex, childbirth may make you looser.

This is because there's never been a penis in history that's as big as a baby.

20. The average vagina produces up to two teaspoons of discharge a day.

But it happens so gradually, it's almost impossible to collect enough at any given time to stir it into your coffee.

21. Like a face, a vagina may sag with age.

The ravages of time may weaken the female genital tract's tautness. To avoid this horrid situation, perform Kegel exercises, don't get fat, and don't smoke.

22. Most nerve vaginal nerve endings are located in the first inch or two of the vaginal opening.

This is why an extremely thick two-inch penis may provide more pleasure than a string-bean-shaped eight-inch penis.

23. "Lady boners" are real.

The clitoris swells and increases in size during female arousal.

24. The clitoris is much larger than what you can see with the naked eye.

Although the visible part of the clitoris is only an inch or so, the rest of it extends within the body for up to six inches.

25. Orgasm is more likely right before or during menstruation.

This seems sort of reproductively counterintuitive, for it would have made more sense if Lord Jehovah had given women more orgasmic capacity during ovulation, but the Lord works in mysterious ways.

CHAPTER 9.

EIGHTEEN SCIENTIFIC REASONS WHY HAVING MORE SEX WILL IMPROVE YOUR ENTIRE LIFE

---

1. It's a proven medical fact that having tons of sex will make you look younger.

Our finest scientists have proved that shagging and shtupping and screwing can prevent the aging process. Sex boots collagen production and releases the human growth hormone. A decade-long study of 3,500 adults in Scotland showed that people who had sex four times a week appeared seven to twelve years younger than their real age. So if you want to look young, get out there and *start fuckin'!*

2. It's a better painkiller than prescription painkillers.

A German study from 2013 found that a majority of migraine sufferers reported partial or total relief after having an orgasm. A study at Rutgers University showed that women's pain tolerance threshold increased 74.6% directly after cumming. "Through sexual arousal and orgasm the hormone oxytocin is secreted in your body, which in turn causes the release of endorphins," says Dr. Desmond Ebanks. "Because of these natural opiates, sex acts as a powerful analgesic." According to sex researcher Stefanie Iris Weiss, "I often tell friends suffering from cramps to go for a sex session rather than an Advil.

3. Your self-esteem will skyrocket.

According to sex researcher Limor Blockman, orgasms release endorphins that improve one's self-perception: "Self-esteem can be easily boosted by the ability to surrender to pleasure and…brag about it…the fact that we allow ourselves to be exposed and enjoy it is a definite, well-proven self-esteem enhancer."

4. It's the best-known stress reliever

throughout recorded human history–and probably into prehistoric times, too.

In stress tests ranging from doing mental arithmetic out loud to public speaking, celibates showed the highest stress levels. Vigorous and frequent sex will flood your brain with endorphins, AKA "the human body's natural heroin."

5. You will sleep better, even if he snores.

A vigorous round of barnyard-animal-level rutting releases super-strong hormones such as vasopressin, oxytocin, and serotonin—which to the human body is like doing a shot of whiskey followed by a beer and then a Xanax. Poof! You're out cold.

6. Your rotten mood will improve, thank God.

All the sex hormones that soak your brain after an orgasm will induce a sense of euphoria and well-being akin to eating an entire box of chocolate while stroking a litter of newborn puppies.

7. Your skin will glow as if you were an angel, a space alien, or an angelic space alien.

Your body produces more collagen as a result of sex, which makes your skin appear as fresh as the morning dew. Women who have more sex also release more estrogen. The result? Happy skin on a happy woman!

8. Your hair will become like the shiniest silk woven by tiny invisible fairies on a divine loom.

The estrogen and testosterone that the body releases during sex help you maintain a shiny mane that would be the envy of any racehorse. Regular sex also allows the body to more efficiently metabolize nutrients, leading to shinier and silkier hair. Go ahead—have a lot of sex and then touch your hair if you don't believe me.

9. It will alleviate your wretched and unjust menstrual suffering.

Uterine contraction during orgasm increases blood flow to the area and relieves cramping. Don't let Aunt Flo deter you—whip out that Magic Wand and get to work!

10. You will be immune to disease, even if you're not immune to criticism.

Having lots of sex increases levels of the anti-body IgA into the bloodstream, bolstering the immune system. Regular sex has also been known protect you against the common cold. So go ahead and take ten minutes to rub one out—it's better than blowing your nose for a week.

11. It burns calories like a blowtorch.

About 25 minutes of sex is all you need to wipe away the 195 calories from that choco-late donut you ate right before he rang your doorbell. If you have sex all night, you might even be able to eat an entire pizza with no ill effects to your waistline.

12. You will become a lean, pristine, fighting machine.

I swapped out the word "mean" for "pristine," because sex will actually cure you of mean-ness. But all the testosterone released during sexual activity will help create lean muscle mass and tone your physique to the point where it will repel bullets.

13. It will turn your frown upside-down.

Numerous studies have proved that semen contains compounds that have antidepressant qualities. One study showed that women who have unprotected sex had lower levels of depression than women who used condoms or didn't have sex at all.

14. Duh! It will make you smarter.

A study on sexually active rats—ew!—showed that they grew extra brain neurons as a result of their bawdy activity. A researcher at the University of Amsterdam used MRIs to conclude that there is "a very widespread increase in the functional brain activity at orgasm." So don't be dumb—have more sex!

15. It even cures the hiccups!

A 2000 report in *Canadian Family Physician* detailed the case of a healthy man who was cured of his chronic hiccups at the moment he ejaculated during intercourse. Hiccups are cured when the vagus nerve is stimulated, which happens during sex.

16. Having oodles of orgasms can protect you against certain forms of cancer.

A French study revealed that women who frequently had intercourse were only one-third as likely to develop breast cancer compared to women who didn't fuck as much. A 2004 National Cancer Institute study of 50,000 men revealed that guys who blew at least 21 loads per month were 30% less likely to get prostate cancer than those poor saps who had seven or fewer orgasms monthly. A 2003 study found than men who had five orgasms a week while in their 20s were one-third less likely to develop prostate cancer later in life.

17. It will keep your heart healthy—which will enable you to have more sex.

A European study found that the more often a man had sex, the lower his blood pressure was. A study in *Journal of Epidemiology and Community Health* concluded that having sex at least twice a week cut one's heart-attack risk in half.

18. You will live longer—which will enable you to have even more sex.

A 1997 *British Medical Journal* study found that men who ejaculated frequently—and what man doesn't like to do that?—had a 50% lower mortality rate than men who didn't. So, gents, for the sake of your family, loved ones, and sundry other dependents—bust a nut and live longer!

CHAPTER 10.

GET BUZZED!: TWENTY LITTLE-KNOWN FACTS ABOUT VIBRATORS

---

1. GOOD FOR YOUR HEALTH

Research has shown that women who use vibrators are more likely to visit the gynecologist for checkups, to achieve orgasm with or without a vibrator, and to have lower stress levels and fewer headaches than women who don't use them. What's not to like?

2. UM, WHERE DO YOU PUT IT?

One study revealed that a whoppin' 83.8% of female vibrator users preferred to employ the device for clitoral stimulation rather than vaginal insertion. But hey, you can put it anywhere you like!

3. A $1 BILLION MARKET

One billion dollars' worth of vibrators are sold every year, accounting for a bigger market even than condoms.

4. A VIBRATOR FOR EVERY NEED

No two vaginas (or anuses) are alike, which is why sex-toy technicians have bequeathed us with a wide, wonderful, throbbing world of vibrators from which to choose. Some types, such as the monstrously sized and monstrously popular Hitachi Magic Wand, are sold as "back massagers" and are intended strictly for clitoral stimulation. Others are shaped like penises and are made for vaginal insertion. Some are waterproof, enabling you to rub one out in the shower or hot tub. The "rabbit" (more on that later) is two-pronged, with the larger prong for vaginal insertion and the smaller one for clitoral stimulation. Some are shaped to stimulate the G-spot or prostate gland. There are even "smart" vibrators than can be programmed over the Internet to include different vibration patterns and music to your self-pleasuring sessions.

5. CLEOPATRA'S ANGRY BEES

As legend has it, Cleopatra, the Queen of Egypt whose seductive powers culminated in the Roman Civil War, invented the hand-held vibrator by filling a hollowed gourd with angry bees and then pressing it against her nether regions. Hail to the Queen Bee!

6. CURING "HYSTERIA"

Back in the Sexual Dark Ages before men realized that women have orgasms, females' pent-up sexual frustration was diagnosed as a medical condition called "hysteria." The cure? Originally, it was a visit to the doctor's office, where a woman would receive a "pelvic massage"—i.e., a handjob—until she had a "hysterical paroxysm," which is now called an orgasm. For eons, physicians used their own hands. But amid the industrial hubbub of the 1800s, inventors coughed up a dizzying area of giant steampunk contraptions designed to cure "hysteria"—some of them required two people to operate them, and a few were even steam-powered.

7. THE FRENCH WIND-UP TOY (1734)

The first "modern" vibrator was a little hand-powered box invented in France and called *le tremoussoir*. You cranked it up like a music box, but instead of playing "Twinkle, Twinkle, Little Star," it gave you an orgasm.

8. THE FIRST ELECTRIC VIBRATOR (1883)

In 1883, British doctor J. Mortimer Granville patented a forty-pound electromechanical monster that was the first modern "hysteria" cure powered by electricity. He quickly became the most popular doctor in England—among women, at least.

9. THE FIRST HAND-HELD PERSONAL VIBRATOR (1902)

These "hysteria" cures became so popular that in 1902, Hamilton Beach patented the first handheld, electro-powered personal vibrator for home use. Vibrators were only the fifth electrical device in history to receive a patent—after the toaster, sewing machine, fan, and tea kettle. American women were using vibrators at home before they were using vacuum cleaners.

10. THE DARK AGES OF MODERN VIBRATORS

By the 1920s, it began slowly dawning on American men that their wives were using electrical vibrators at home for sexual gratification. *That's* how slow they were back then! This led to an outright ban on vibrators that lasted all the way until the late 1960s. The prohibition on alcohol, which started around the same time as the prohibition on vibrators, only lasted 11 years. But vibrators were banned for at least 40 years. Get your priorities straight, Americans!

11. THE CORDLESS REVOLUTION

Amid the social tumult of the 1960s came the Sexual Revolution. One of the primary tools of this revolution, along with birth-control pills, was the cordless personal vibrator. In 1968, a patent was issued for a "Cordless Electric Vibrator for Use on the Human Body," and the buzzing has never stopped.

12. LOUD VIBRATIONS FROM DOWN UNDER

You may think of New Zealand as Australia's homely little sister, but the Pacific island nation has the world's highest rate of vibrator ownership—38% of Kiwis own a vibrator.

13. DON'T BELIEVE THE STEREOTYPE

Contrary to stereotypes that women use vibrators because they can't snag a living penis, one study showed that four out of every five female vibrator users was in a relationship.

14. MOST MEN ARE NOT THREATENED BY THEM

Despite the popular notion that men experience severe castration anxiety and fear of mechanical cuckoldry whenever they see a vibrator, one study showed that seven out of ten men were absolutely A-OK with their lady friends using vibrators.

15. VIBRATOR-INDUCED HOSPITAL VISITS

In 2014, a Kansas woman was rushed to the hospital because a tiny, pinkie-sized vibrator got caught in her urethra and managed to vibrate itself all the way up to her bladder. In 2013, a man live-tweeted his hospital visit for getting a vibrating dildo stuck up his rectum.

16. ALABAMA: NO VIBRATORS FOR YOU!

Alabama's Anti-Obscenity Enforcement Act bans the sale of "any device designed or marketed as useful for the stimulation of human genital organs." If you want to get a vibrator in Alabama, you'll need a doctor's note.

17. MORE RELIGION = FEWER VIBRATORS

Religious belief is negatively correlated with vibrator ownership, but you probably already suspected that.

18. SILLY RABBIT!

The two-pronged "rabbit" vibrator, made famous in an episode of *Sex and the City*, contains a phallic prong and a smaller prong that directly stimulates the clitoris. It was initially designed in Japan to look like a rabbit because of a Japanese law forbidding the sale of items that look like penises. According to some, it is now the world's biggest-selling sex toy.

19. THE $55,000 VIBRATOR

The world's priciest sex toy is fashioned from white gold and is covered in 117 diamonds. The cost? A highly reasonable $55,000.

20. MEET "BOB"

That's an acronym for "Battery-Operated Boyfriend." If you can come up with a cuter name for your vibrator, go for it!

CHAPTER 11.

TWENTY-FIVE FACTS ABOUT SEMEN

---

1. Semen is much, much more than just sperm.

Although many people use the words "sperm" and "semen" as if they were synonymous, how tragically wrong these mortal fools are! The truth is that sperm comprises only about 5-10% of any given male jizzload. The rest is comprised of rich, happy bodily fluids and a dazzling array of nutrients that aid, protect, and comfort the sperm in its long and arduous journey toward the haughty female egg.

2. Semen is so chock-full of nutrients, it's a wonder that people don't eat more of it.

Semen contains vitamin C, fructose, magnesium, phosphorus, potassium, vitamin B12, zinc, nitrogen, and calcium. The average male jizzwad is said to contain roughly as much protein as an egg white (chicken, not human eggs, of course). And all this life-giving nutrition will only set your diet back 20 calories!

3. The average size of a male jizzload is half a teaspoon.

Every male who's reading this is grabbing a teaspoon and desperately checking to see how he measures up to others.

4. There are around 200 million sperm in an average human jizzload.

That's roughly the same number of sperm in the average rabbit jizzload. The mighty pig, however, shoots out nearly eight billion little piggy wrigglers with every foul porcine orgasm.

5. Sperm take about 75 days to grow in the testes.

Just as men are always expected to be making money, they are always making sperm, too—roughly 1,500 every second. On average, these rambunctious li'l critters spend two and a half months developing inside a man's scrotum before he suddenly murders them by the hundreds of millions during one wanton jack-off session to some online porn of questionable taste.

6. Sperm can live for up to five days inside a vagina, depending on how friendly the vagina is.

On average, sperm live about 24-48 hours once inside the human vagina. If the host female's acidic balance is propitious, sperm can live up to five days inside her womb before perishing. In contrast, bat sperm can live up to 145 days, which should make every bat who's reading this feel incredibly macho.

7. Sperm that is not ejaculated gets broken down and reabsorbed into the body.

If a man has an inactive sex life and can't even be bothered to pleasure himself, sperm that stores up inside his body without being released will eventually die and be reabsorbed into his body like so much horse manure spread judiciously throughout a cornfield.

8. Men never stop making semen.

Although women stop producing eggs after

menopause, men continue creating sperm and seminal fluid up until the day they croak. Science currently offers no answers regarding what happens to semen in the afterlife. It is not known whether semen exists in heaven, although it's highly likely there's plenty of semen in hell.

9. Good diet = good sperm.

Sperm count and quality can be greatly affected by a man's dietary habits. Foods that will give you vibrant, healthy, muscular, happy, robust sperm include oysters, bananas, walnuts, asparagus, garlic, lean beef, and chocolate. It's also important to drink plenty of water, because sperm spend their brief lives pretty much submerged in a swimming pool of your balls' own making.

10. Bad diet = bad sperm.

If you want a healthy baby, put down the cigarettes and bongs, stay away from the vodka, say "no" to the bacon, cheese, cupcakes, and sausages, and drink decaf. That's if you want a healthy baby—I didn't say anything about having a happy life.

11. Some people use semen in their cooking recipes.

Well, at least one person does. This mysterious Semen Chef's name is "Fotie Photenhauer," and this shadowy person of dubious name and indeterminate gender has released a book called *Natural Harvest: a collection of semen-based recipes*.

From the book's online description:

> Semen is not only nutritious, but it also has a wonderful texture and amazing cooking properties. Like fine wine and cheeses, the taste of semen is complex and dynamic. Semen is inexpensive to produce and is commonly available in many, if not most, homes and restaurants.

12. Obesity lowers sperm count and quality.

Gents, if your BMI is 25 or above, allow me to loudly ring the alarm bell and inform you that your sperm will be slower, fewer in number, and less capable of winning a Gold Medal in swimming than the sperm of slimmer men. What you choose to do about this fact is between you and your so-called "God."

13. Most sperm are abnormal.

That's right—"abnormal." I didn't say "weird." I didn't say that anyone should bully them. Many sperm are born with two heads or two tails. Sometimes their heads range in size from puny to enormous. Sometimes their tails are crooked. According to one website, "90% of sperm ejaculated are deformed." So in this case, the "normal" ones are the "weird" ones.

14. Most sperm can't even swim straight.

Upon being ejaculated into a moist and willing vagina, only about one in five sperm even have the basic common sense to start swimming upstream toward the female's egg. Others will swim in circles. Yet others will simply tread water.

15. Sperm are either male or female.

Sperm will either carry a female "X" chromosome or a male "Y" chromosome—not both—which will eventually determine the baby's sex. Male sperm allegedly swim faster, but female sperm are said to be stronger during that long, deadly *Heart of Darkness*-styled ride upstream toward the egg.

16. Those li'l tadpoles like it cold.

The main reason you have a scrotum in the first place is so that people can make fun of the word "scrotum." The second reason you have a scrotum is that healthy sperm enjoy temperatures about seven degrees lower than the average human body temperature, so they like to "chill" by hanging in that disgusting little skin hammock between your legs. Men also produce more sperm in the winter than in the summer.

17. Those li'l tadpoles die when it gets hot.

If you spend too much time in hot tubs, you will effectively turn your sperm into hundreds of millions of boiled eggs, rendering you sterile—if that's your idea of a good time. It can also lower your sperm count for up to six months. The condition is known as "scrotal hyperthermia." Other instances of sperm-death-by-overheating can be caused by tight underwear and putting your laptop…in…your…lap.

18. Some women are allergic to semen.

The condition is known as "seminal plasma

hypersensitivity" and can cause redness, swelling, itching, and burning in the vaginal area. It doesn't mean she doesn't like you. It only means that her body hates your sperm.

19. Semen makes a good cosmetic.

A compound in semen known as "spermine" is an antioxidant known to smooth wrinkles and alleviate acne. Spermine is featured in cosmetic creams offered by several swanky high-end spas to the tune of about $250 per tube. Surely there are more natural and frugal methods to obtain spermine? Whatever could they be?

20. Semen has antidepressant qualities.

Semen contains dozens of compounds that that have all been known to alleviate the psychological malady known as "the blues." Semen is a mood-enhancing potion that contains cortisol, estrone, oxytocin, prolactin, melatonin, and serotonin.

21. Dead sperm can still fertilize an egg.

In laboratory settings, scientists have been able to fertilize female human eggs using dead human sperm. Apparently the DNA, dead or alive, is all that's needed to start bakin' a baby.

22. Frequent ejaculation improves sperm quality.

Even if you don't want to reproduce, there is no reasonable or justifiable excuse for not ejaculating as frequently as possible, even if you're forced to take matters into your own hands.

23. British spies in World War I used semen as invisible ink.

No, I'm not kidding. And the name of the high-ranking military-intelligence official who ordered a study on whether semen would make an effective invisible ink was "Mansfield Cumming."

24. Wireless technology can damage sperm.

It's not only the heat from a toasty laptop that can kill or harm your sperm—the very WiFi connection that allows you to post on Facebook twenty thousand times a day can potentially harm both sperm and eggs. Radiofrequency electromagnetic waves are thought to induce oxidative damage to both sperm and eggs.

25. It only takes one ball to get the ball rolling.

If you have only one testicle—like, say, you're Lance Armstrong—you can still produce enough healthy sperm to reproduce.

CHAPTER 12.

SEVENTEEN OF THE WACKIEST MYTHS & TABOOS ABOUT MENSTRUATION YOU'VE EVER HEARD

---

1. Don't go into the ocean when you have your period, because sharks will attack you.

According to a scientific study wherein sharks were exposed to various human bodily fluids, the only one that attracted them was a specific stomach acid. So as long as you don't vomit into the water, you should be cool.

2. Don't go into the woods, either, because the bears can smell your menstruation.

The bears are only concerned about whether you've brought along sandwiches.

3. Don't go into the fields, either, because you'll kill all the crops.

According to Roman naturalist Pliny the Elder:

> Contact with the monthly flux of women turns new wine sour, makes crops wither, kills grafts, dries seeds in gardens, causes the fruit of trees to fall off, dims the bright surface of mirrors, dulls the edge of steel and the gleam of ivory, kills bees, rusts iron and bronze, and causes a horrible smell to fill the air. Dogs who taste the blood become mad, and their bite becomes poisonous as in rabies. The Dead Sea, thick with salt, cannot be drawn asunder except by a thread soaked in the poisonous fluid of the menstruous blood. A thread from an infected dress is sufficient. Linen, touched by the woman while boiling and washing it in water, turns black.

Holy shit, dude. Pardon me for thinking you may have had problem that extended far beyond having to deal with menstrual blood.

4. Sex during menstruation can yield deformed or red-haired babies.

It's possible to get pregnant during your period, but there is no evidence it will lead to birth defects or red hair, not that the two are related.

5. Babies conceived during a woman's period will be "monsters."

At least that's according to old French folk-lore. But the French also rolled over for Hitler and think that Jerry Lewis is a genius, so take everything they say with a grain of salt.

6. Don't drink any menstrual blood, because you might contract leprosy.

So go ahead—chug menstrual blood by the gallon. Unless it came from a leper, you're cool—no risk of leprosy.

7. Hanging a sack full of ashes from a burnt toad near your coochie will alleviate a heavy flow.

Such was the common wisdom in medieval Europe. It seems more likely that burnt-toad ashes would alleviate vaginal lubrication as well as killing every erection within a hundred yards, but what do I know?

8. Menstrual blood can turn wine into vinegar.

This was a common myth in Europe a few centuries ago. Presumably after the wine was turned into vinegar they called in Jesus, who turned it back into wine.

7. If you received dental fillings during your period, they will fall out of your mouth.

If, say, the dental fillings were to fall out of your mouth, chances are close to 100% that it had to do more with your dentist than with your period.

8. Dough will refuse to rise if a menstruating woman is on a bakery's premises.

This presumes that dough is a sentient being capable of being aware that a woman is on the bakery's premises—a shaky presumption, to be sure. But it was alleged in the 1920s by a Viennese scientist named Bela Schick.

9. Menstrual blood contains poisons known as "menotoxins."

That same Viennese scientist theorized that "menotoxins" were a poison contained in menstrual fluid that so powerful it could cause flowers to wilt. I'd like to tell him that he was wrong, but it's likely that his flower wilted long ago.

10. Do NOT wash your hair while on your period—*period.*

Not only will you cause your hair to lose its natural body and bounce, it can cause health problems all the way up to and including cancer.

11. Slipping some of your period blood into a man's food or drink will cause him to fall madly in love with you.

This is a common misconception across several African and Asian cultures. I suppose the key is that you never *tell* your suitor you've spiked his food or beverage with your period blood, because it'll likely gross him out.

12. Menstrual blood can ward off demons.

Everyone on Earth knows that the exact opposite is true.

13. A man should never come into contact with menstrual blood, because it will "dull his wits and lead to a slow death."

This is according to folklore in Papua New Guinea, where the guys apparently find it difficult dealing with their girlfriends' monthly visitor. I can't even imagine how they deal with their mothers-in-law.

14. You can contract gonorrhea by having sex with a menstruating woman.

True—but only if she already has gonorrhea.

15. Menstrual fluids are so dirty and foul that they can even rot pickled foods.

The idea that period blood is "unclean" or "dirty" spans almost all global cultures, but in rural India, it's thought to be so toxic that it can cause the humble pickle to rot horribly.

16. Women on their period should be kept far away from the public water supply lest they contaminate it.

This is a myth common in several Southeast Asian communities. The only way that menstruating women would contaminate the local water supply is if they purposely put poison in it to publish a community so stupid and backward that it thinks menstrual fluids are Satan's blood.

17. Menstrual blood mixed with wine and sprinkled over a field will help crops to grow.

At least that's what the ancient Greeks thought—probably at a moment when they were mixing everything with wine.

CHAPTER 13.

TWENTY-FIVE LITTLE-KNOWN FACTS ABOUT YOUR PERIOD

---

1. It's a biological fact that menstruating makes you less attractive to men.

A man's testosterone levels are directly affected by a woman's scent, which changes during a menstrual cycle. One study where men sniffed the T-shirts of women who were ovulating showed the men's testosterone levels spike, while testosterone decreased when they sniffed T-shirts of women who weren't ovulating. Another study showed that strippers make *twice* as much in tips when they're ovulating than when they're on their period.

2. It's also a biological fact that menstruating makes you hornier.

The hormone progesterone is said to lower a woman's libido. Yet while menstruating women produce less progesterone, which makes them likelier to crave sex during this phase.

3. The average total amount of blood lost during a period is anywhere from two tablespoons to half a cup.

The average amount of blood lost during a menstrual phase is around three tablespoons. This includes blood clots. Any blood loss totaling a cup or more could be the sign of a serious medical problem.

4. Women in Western cultures will experience about 450 periods over their lifetime.

This stands in contrast to prehistoric women, who only menstruated about 50 times over the course of their lives. It also contrasts with modern women in agrarian regions, who only menstruate about 150 times total. The inescapable conclusion is that capitalism and

Western civilization lead to increased menstruation.

5. The average woman will spend nearly ten years of her life menstruating.

In other words, about 3,500 days of the average woman's life will be spent "on the rag."

6. The average woman will use nearly 11,000 tampons over her lifetime.

You could build a house with that many used tampons, although it's probably not advisable.

7. You can use tampons and still be a virgin.

Since tampons are thankfully smaller and thinner than most penises, a girl can safely insert one inside her vagina without rupturing her hymen. Besides, one loses one's virginity by having sex, not by breaking their hymen.

8. Most girls get their first period around age 12.

It varies of course, but the age of 12 is an average launching pad for a girl and her period pads. She will continue menstruating until around age 50.

9. In olden days, girls didn't used to get their first period until around age 16 or 17.

In the 1800s, the average girl did not get her first period until well into her teens. It is thought that girls reach puberty earlier these days due to a combination of better nutrition and increased stress.

10. It is perfectly normal to have irregular periods up until about age 18.

It usually takes girls a few years before their menstrual cycle settles into a regular pattern. Early menstrual cycles can be very short (21 days) or very long (45 days), but they usually even out around the age of 18.

11. The average menstrual cycle is slightly shorter than one month.

Although it is commonly believed that a woman's cycle is determined by the monthly phases of the moon, on average it lasts about 28-29 days—which makes it perfect for February but a little short for all other months.

12. Women experience more brutal periods during the colder months.

A period's pain level, blood flow, and duration tend to be longer during the winter months than in summer.

13. Science still doesn't know whether it's true that women who live together wind up synchronizing their periods.

Although many women swear that they always wind up having their periods around the same time as their close friends, science has yet to definitively answer whether this legend is true.

14. Menstrual discharge contains more than blood.

It also contains shedded uterine tissue, which gives it a thicker and gummier consistency than blood alone.

15. Your period can also change your voice.

One study published in the journal *Ethology* claimed that men who listened to recordings of women's voices were generally able to tell which women were menstruating. One would assume that their tone while menstruating was slightly more menacing than normal.

16. You can still get pregnant on your period.

It's unlikely, but still possible, since sperm can stay alive inside the vagina for up to a week. The risk of pregnancy is highest when having sex during the end of one's menstrual cycle.

17. If you're bleeding, that may be a sign of pregnancy rather than menstruation.

Just because you're bleeding doesn't mean it's your period. During the early stages of pregnancy, women may experience light blood flow or spotting due to a process known as "implantation bleeding."

18. Your body mimics the symptoms of pregnancy in the days leading up to your period.

In the days leading up to when Aunt Flo knocks on the door, your body secretes hormones that cause irritability, feeling bloated, acne, and fluid retention—which are precisely the same symptoms one experiences during pregnancy.

19. Human females are one of the only mammals that go through menopause.

The other two breeds are elephants and humpback whales.

20. PMS can make you more violent.

One study of female prison inmates concluded that they are far more likely to commit violent acts in the days preceding menstruation than in the days directly after menstruation.

21. You may think more like a male while you're menstruating.

Lowered estrogen levels during menstruation may actually enhance a woman's "male cognitive skills," lending a temporary cognitive advantage in areas such as spatial thinking.

22. Your period can cause an iron deficiency.

Losing all that blood means losing all that iron. You may also feel so rotten and fatigued, you don't bother ironing your clothes.

23. You need a little bit of body fat in order to menstruate.

If your body fat plummets below 8-12%, your period will abruptly cease, if it ever began at all. Fat cells are correlated with a woman's estrogen levels and are thus necessary in both menstruation and procreation.

24. Menstrual symptoms lead to 100 million lost work hours in America yearly.

It's a legitimate medical excuse, one that men are never able to claim.

25. While menstruating, you may bleed from places other than your vagina.

In a very rare medical condition known as "vicarious menstruation," women on their period may also harmlessly bleed from their mouth, ears, lungs, nose, eyes, and skin. It is not known exactly why this happens, only that it does.

ABOUT THE AUTHOR

Lorenzo Jensen III is the son and grandson of two men who thought they were so great, they cloned themselves. He enjoys skeet-shooting, kite-flying, and wrestling naked with pit bulls. He writes about sex because he never has any.